BREAKUP to MAKEUP:

Getting Your "Ex" Back

Introduction

I have been counseling women of all ages, religions, races and occupations for more than 20 years. In this time I have found that very few, if any, were prepared for the dissolution of a relationship commonly called a "breakup". Whether it was a marriage, a long or short-term relationship or even an infatuation I found that women were unable to move forward and literally became emotionally paralyzed by the event. There is nothing that leaves you feeling less powerful than being dumped by a man! It is this feeling of abandonment and helplessness that drives women to do crazy things that push the guy away even more. Don't let this happen to you!

A break-up is as devastating as a death and just about as hard to get over. It can totally destroy a woman's self-confidence and I have seen it take years to fully recover in the absence of help from an outsider. As a relationship counselor it has been my duty and privilege to guide and empower women in every area of their lives. Having been there myself I know the difficulties of facing a life without the person you dreamed of being by your side. I also know how to get him back as you grow stronger and stronger each day. Being so empowered that you will not actually "need" him to make you feel whole and purposeful. He will be an addition to your happy life and your world will no longer revolve around him.

If you find yourself facing an emotional challenge, such as the unexpected loss of your mate's love, this book will help to empower you and move forward with your life. There is nothing positive that can be accomplished by sitting around mourning the loss of someone and possibly doing the *exact opposite* of what should be done to win the person back, if they even deserve to be in your life again, and that is something only you can decide. Take a positive step today and allow me to guide you to the "new you". The strong, positive, independent, wonderful woman that every man desires – not just the "ex" you want to attract.

This is the fourth book in my best selling "FOR WOMEN ONLY" series that was created to help my sisters excel in love. Enjoy!

He Loved You Once & He Will Love You Again….if you play your cards right!

"The most painful thing is losing yourself in the process of loving someone too much, and forgetting that you are special too." -- Ernest Hemingway

If you are newly single, or newly dumped, you are probably going over and over in your mind the beginning of your relationship and just how magical it was. Wondering what went wrong and remembering all of the little things that he did, said or expressed and missing him like crazy. You most likely didn't see this coming and were blindsided by the breakup. Even if it has happened to you before with the same person, and there is a pattern of instability, you most likely were not prepared for it to happen again. Torturing yourself with repetitive negative thoughts isn't going to bring him back or make you stronger. It will end up being destructive to you and your future with your "ex".

Asking yourself: "What went wrong? Why did he leave? Does he still love me?" These are all normal questions, and understandable, but the questions are futile because it doesn't really matter. There is absolutely nothing you can do to change the past no matter how much time and energy you waste by focusing on it! Projecting into the future with statements like these may sabotage your relationship and make you feel totally helpless: "Can I get him back? Is he with someone else? How can I live without him?" You can begin today to change the outcome of a breakup and that is what you will begin doing immediately with the help of a few simple, yet effective exercises.

If your man loved you, desired you or had *ANY* feelings toward you whatsoever you can ignite them again. That's the good news! You have a distinct advantage over all other females he comes into contact with because he has already given his heart to you -- once. Therefore, giving it to you again will be easier and faster if you work quickly to take control of the situation and your emotions.

I am assuming that the "ex" is someone who is worthy of your time, attention and affection. If he were a serial cheater, an abuser or a player I wouldn't waste my time on getting him back. I would simply realize that I dodged a bullet and move on in my life. However, if he was a "quality man" and you still love him then these steps will increase the likelihood that he will return but as an even better mate than before.

First of all, you must ask yourself whether he broke up with you in a manner befitting your relationship. A woman I counseled was in an "on again – off again" relationship for 9 years with a man who would simply disappear when he got bored and decided he wanted to chase someone new. After being with him this last time for 8 months he left the country for a vacation with another woman and didn't even bother to tell Kathy he was going. It was only by accident she found out and when he returned he didn't bother to contact her for another two months! When he did contact her he acted as if nothing was different between the two of them. Unforgivable behavior like this should not be tolerated and she should never allow this man back into her life no matter how much she loves him and with my assistance she won't succumb to his charm again.

Why? He has proven that he has no respect for her or her feelings and he is not ever going to change. He knew he hurt her when he did the same thing numerous times but he never changed his behavior. Why waste more time on someone who is not a good choice for a mate? She desires someone she can count on and he has proven time and time again that he is not that person. If he loved her and respected her, even as a friend, he would not abuse their relationship the way he has.

How your man breaks up with you says a lot about his character. A "real man" will sit down with you face-to-face and explain why he does not want to continue the relationship. A man who is a selfish narcissist and has no respect for you will disappear only to re-appear when he has satisfied his needs and selfish desires elsewhere and wants the comfort and safety of your relationship and love. In other words he is not interested in a long-term relationship and only seeks out comfort and love when he desires it and he does not concern himself with your needs. A man who will send you a text message to breakup is a coward and thinks very little of the relationship. The way he breaks it off will speak volumes about him as a person and as a potential lifetime mate.

If your man loves and respects you, but doesn't see a future whatever the reasons may be, he will explain his reason for breaking up in person. Those men are worth the energy and effort necessary to get them back. Whatever the reasons were for the breakup they loved you once and they can love you again. You can get the relationship to be even stronger than before if you don't blow it by making all the mistakes women generally make before you get the chance to reconcile.

Even if he broke up because he is infatuated with another woman, or simply wants his freedom, you can keep yourself on his mind and in his heart if you follow a few simple rules. I broke up with Allen after a very intense, powerful love connection that I had never experienced before. It felt, at the time, like we were *soulmates*. You know, that catchy phrase that women want to call the person who seems to be everything they desire in life and more. He was extremely handsome, passionate and a good lover, was wealthy, attentive and the man of my dreams....until he wasn't. One day after a slight disagreement with me he slept with his "ex" and I booted him to the curb immediately. He wasn't worthy of my love and affection. I didn't want to spend time trying to change a man who had no morals and no respect for me as a person. A *soulmate* would not behave the way he did and I recognized that he was not the person I created in my mind.

Could I have attracted him back? Of course! He begged, cried and pleaded for reconciliation but I didn't want to ignite the love and passion because he was a man who was unworthy of it. He had proven to me that he was untrustworthy and I am wise enough to know that people do not fundamentally change. It was not in my best interest to hang onto a relationship knowing how it would end. After all, he cheated on me with his "ex" and before me I found out that he cheated on his "ex" with others. A pattern was there that was undeniable and, as hurt as I was over the breakup, I healed very quickly because I knew he wasn't the man of my dreams. I knew I deserved better!

My point in telling you this story is because if there is a pattern there that cannot be denied don't think you can change the person to suit you. Read this book to assist you in being a stronger woman, an empowered person, a woman who attracts what she desires and one that men desire but not to get that nasty "ex" back! You will find the more you do things for yourself the more you attract quality men. The stronger you are and the higher your self-esteem the less you will want a man who doesn't love and respect you.

Now let's get back to the subject of getting your love back in your arms. I will use my favorite restaurant as an analogy of your relationship with your love because there is a restaurant that I go to regularly and I love it. Why? Because it feels like home away from home and it gives me great comfort the moment I walk in the front door. I know the staff, I am greeted by name, I always have a special place to sit and I know a lot of the regulars. It is familiar and it makes me feel comfortable and secure. Do I go to other restaurants? Of course! I love trying out new places and experiencing different things but this place is one of a kind special to me.

It is the same with your "ex". You have a familiar relationship. It is comforting to him to not have to be someone he isn't when trying to impress other women. He is no different from you in that no one likes to be actively seeking a relationship and it gets tiresome very fast. It requires time, money and going through a lot of crazy women to find one who may fit into a narrowly defined category of *possible* mates. It may seem like an adventure at first but it quickly turns into a nightmare of disappointments and failures.

Let's take my restaurant example. What if it closed? It's my safe place and it would be devastating if I could never go back there, which I invariably do. Just the thought that it may go away makes me want to go there more frequently. Your relationship is basically the same thing. Later in the book I will explain the reasons you will go into a no contact mode after the breakup and this is just one of the reasons.

Missing you is extremely important! The thought of you not being there, even as a backup plan, is frightening to him.

When he goes out with his friends, meets new women and/or even goes out on a date he doesn't forget about the intimacy he shared with you. In fact, play your cards right and every woman will be up against his memory of you. That's pretty powerful because you, and only you, have a special *love place* in his heart so it is 10 times easier for you to get him back instead of lose him entirely. Just like my restaurant example I may stray and try something new, but it will not be easily replaced and I will be eager to go back to the welcoming environment.

Only you and your man know what happened that broke the two of you apart but I am telling you that unless you pulled out a gun and threatened to shoot him he still has positive thoughts about you and your relationship. I know a woman who actually did threaten to kill her man with a loaded gun and he still took her back so I can confirm that positive feelings do not go away easily.

Why do you think people who reunite at a high school reunion frequently begin their relationship again just like 20 years had not gone by? The passion and love that was once there is easily reignited even after years and years of no contact! You and your mate have each created an image in your mind of each other that is not easily destroyed. In fact, whatever happened between you, even if it was a monstrous breakup, will not easily kill the love.

You have an advantage that no one else has with your "ex" because you are the *most recent* memory of love and companionship that he can recall. It will be difficult for someone else to penetrate the barrier and essence of *YOU* that is literally and figuratively all over him. Unless you go nuts and destroy the ties you have to one another there is an excellent chance you will end up together and happy. It is not too late for you to become the woman he will never want to leave. When you have respect and love for yourself you will teach him the boundaries that he will learn to honor and respect. It is you that allowed him to treat you poorly and it will be you that will make him *WANT* to treat you differently.

If you are not getting what you desire out of relationship it is because you set your expectations too low and allowed someone to treat you disrespectfully. A woman who values herself will never allow anyone -- whether it is a man, woman or child -- to treat them badly. Low self-esteem is generally the cause of accepting less than you deserve or desire but we will address that issue later in the book. It will sabotage your relationship if you let it! Men will treat you the way you train them to treat you! Take that a step further and you will see that you actually train everyone you meet as to what you will and will not accept from them.

Knowing this one simple fact will hopefully make you want to change the way you present yourself to others and change what you are willing to accept from them. Allowing your man to treat you casually and like he could live without you as easily as live with you is unacceptable in every way. You are not an option if you want a connection that leads to marriage and commitment.

It is time to get your man back but on your terms! No more losing yourself in the relationship and giving until you have nothing more to give! A relationship requires work from both parties and you should never be willing to sacrifice your desires and happiness for someone else. A man will not appreciate you any more if you give 99% and he gives 1%. In fact, he will seek out and find someone who requires him to give more than his share to make the union work. Men may push the boundaries but they do so wanting you to show them there is a limit and consequences for their actions.

Why No Contact Works and When To Use It

"Whenever you're in conflict with someone, there is one factor that can make the difference between damaging your relationship and deepening it. That factor is attitude." - *William James*

Let's look at the facts for a moment and maybe you can relate to the reasons behind the "no contact rule". You have just broken up and maybe you feel that you need an opportunity to present your side of the situation to win him back. You were just misunderstood and if you call, text, email or stalk him surely he will see why he should come running back to you. Really? The person who wants nothing to do with you at the moment, and proved it by leaving, will change his mind if you chase him down and force him to reconsider his decision?

You are not going to convince him you are worthy of his love and affection by forcing him to take you back. You aren't going to guilt him into making the decision to take you back. You aren't going to convince him of your worth by tooting your own horn and telling him how great you are and how he will never find another woman like you. What you will do is reinforce his decision to break it off in the first place. Your worth cannot be forced down his throat for him to see that you are the best thing he's ever had in his life. Your absence may make him miss you, desire you and want you back *IF* you are silent in the *correct* way. If you want him to miss you and want you then allow the disconnection. In fact, one of my bestselling meditations is called "Cutting the Cord" and women report amazing things happen when they disconnect from their "ex". It gives the "ex" an opportunity to feel the loss of you and it is important that he does! Something I heartily recommend to everyone going through a breakup.

Immediately after a breakup he knows you are upset and feeling a little crazy and the only thing on his mind is how to avoid contact with you. He doesn't want the drama associated with you and at the moment he may believe he will never want you back. But together we are going to change his mind! I have never encountered a smooth break-up between normal, passionate couples. In fact, it is so disruptive and heart wrenching for the women I have counseled it brings their crazy out even if they are normally sane women. Therefore, it is the worst time to contact him because you will drive him further away than ever.

If you will allow yourself to grieve the loss of him while maintaining sanity **AND** no contact you will be taking the first step to winning his love and affection back. He will be relieved at first to not have to deal with you and the drama he expects. Then after a while, a few days or weeks, he will begin to wonder whether or not you are okay. He will be curious as to why you haven't followed the path of pestering him as he expected. Was he wrong about how important he was in your life? Could it be that your world didn't revolve around him as he thought? Maybe he's not all he thought he was and this idea will begin to affect his self-esteem as he questions his own desirability.

In fact, he may reach out to you to make sure you are miserable and longing for him, as he had hoped. When he does you must reply to his message in a friendly manner but don't jump up and run to him or allow him to see your pain. You are a strong, confident woman and you aren't falling to pieces or check yourself into a mental hospital. It didn't work out but you are fine with the outcome and are moving on. That's the person you are going to project and you are going to "fake it till you make it" and that attitude will actually become how you view the relationship.

If you cry, moan and tell him how much you miss him, how you have wanted to contact him, how lonely and miserable you are, how much you want him back at all costs, and tell him you are willing to do absolutely anything to get him back, he will move on with all the power and self-confidence in the world *AND* it will be without you. Please do not make the mistake of sharing your inner most thoughts and feelings because it will not strengthen you or your relationship with him. This is important to your reconnection with him!

Do not contact him and when he contacts you I want you to be in charge and in control. Does that mean you are a bitch to him? No, absolutely not! You weren't one at the beginning of your relationship otherwise he wouldn't have fallen for you. Men really do not like bitches but bitches do intrigue them for a short period of time. No, you are the confident woman you were when he met you and he needs to prove he is worthy of your love again. You aren't jumping up and down with joy that the man who broke your world apart is now touching base to make sure you are still miserable without him.

No contact works for you because he cannot know without a doubt what is going on in your world and your thoughts. He is just as curious about what you are doing as you are about what he is up to. He will wonder if you are out having fun, lying in bed with a half gallon of ice cream wallowing in self-pity, if guys are busting down your door for dates – all the things you are curious about him he will be about you. Now do you really want to ruin his focus on you by confirming that as badly as you were treated you still can't move forward? No! Absolutely not!

You know what I did when I broke up with someone or they broke it off with me? I deleted their phone numbers, threw away all the cards they gave me, took photos down or deleted them, threw anything they left at my home in the trash, blocked them from social media and erased them from my life. Of course I cried and was sad but I didn't allow them to control my life! I deleted their phone numbers so I couldn't call them if I wanted to because I never memorized the phone numbers. No calls, no texts, no stalking! I did use my secret technique on them to contact them and control their thoughts as I taught you in my first best selling relationship book "Pussy Whip" but that's the ONLY thing I did to contact them. The technique is so powerful and life altering it is the only thing I needed to do!

Another reason not to give in to your weakness and contact them? What you believe will happen is that when they hear your voice it will make them weak in the knees and they will drive like a maniac to get to you and beg for your forgiveness before making out of control passionate love to you. That's what you would do right? Well I have never seen that happen. You have to trust me here, sisters. Not only does that not happen it will delay a positive response and reconciliation. The exact opposite of what you were hoping will happen.

Contacting him will make you weak in his eyes. You will lose the ground you gained when you were in no contact mode. Not because it is a game that you are playing but because it takes the mystery away. Most of the time this is what happens when you contact him.

- He is distant, preoccupied or resolute about the breakup

- You end up being upset, crying or are a bitch to him

- The reason you called or texted is lame and you both know it

- When the call ends it takes you days or weeks to get back to the positive space you were in before it

- The response you got was the exact opposite of what you were hoping and praying for so you're devastated

- Your self-esteem is trashed and the negativity takes over your life pushing him further away

- It re-opens your wounds and it takes that much longer to heal

- You may end up settling for crumbs from him when you could have the whole cake!

In other words it is the worst thing you could have done. I beg you and plead with you not to do it! Is it okay to contact him for his birthday? No! For your anniversary or "special" date to remind him? No! For holidays like Christmas, New Year's or God forbid Valentine's Day? Hell no! There is no occasion that you should contact him and no reason is good enough to pick up your phone. If he left something at your house either throw it away (the immature way) or place it in a box and put it in a closet or the garage. If he wants or needs it he will contact you to get whatever it is.

You and I both know that you are racking your brain to figure out a way to contact him where he won't know that it was planned. Trust me he knows! Everyone knows the story of my fiancé' and I and the fact that we were in a no contact mode for one entire year. Neither of us contacted the other, we didn't run into one another and we were not connected on social media. It was like our relationship never existed. However, I did use my secret technique to send him messages and he never forgot about me, never stopped desiring me and never wanted to. He could not move on without me and that's what you want!

Ladies, it hurts and you feel abandonment and jealousy because you're normal but facing rejection by contacting him is even worse. He needs to cool down and miss you. He needs to pursue you again and *FEEL* what he has lost. He needs to also see you as a woman of character and value and that will happen when you walk away with your head held high. That will happen when he begins to wonder what the hell happened to you and why he didn't make enough of an impact to rock your world.

In a previous book I wrote about a woman who was holding onto a man's leg crying and screaming for him not to leave her. They were in a beautiful, exclusive 5 star resort and she made a spectacle of herself. She didn't get the guy back but he will definitely always have a mental picture of her as he shook her off of his leg. A strong woman is a desirable woman and a man hates drama and chaos more than just about anything in life. Any endearment this man felt for the woman he was with for a few years was erased when she acted as she did and he never went back to her. Her worth was diminished and he didn't see her as a quality woman of value.

Do you know what a man strives for in a relationship? That feeling that he gets right after he has an orgasm where the world is calm, peaceful, loving, uncomplicated and where he is spent, relaxed and without a care in the world. That's what he craves in a relationship and I doubt that's what he had because he probably would not be gone if he did. I'm not busting your chops for not being that woman because really that woman doesn't exist! It's a fanciful notion that he thinks is possible but in reality it is not. It will not be you, or any woman, that can provide that to him but sometimes he needs to figure that out for himself!

However, you can achieve something almost as wonderful if you take away the drama from your relationship. If you take away the stress and pressure and let him miss you. If you realize that you cannot "sell" yourself to him and make him want to be with you. But you can be the high quality, special, desirable woman that he chooses to be with and *THAT* will get him to come back to you.

So what if he doesn't contact you? Well, I will be honest and say that it is not necessarily a sign that he doesn't care. It could be a game that he is playing. My fiancé admits that he never thought we would stay apart but it took a year of no contact for us to get back together. Sometimes there has been so much pain and heartache between the two of you that he may feel you are done and the relationship is over. Are you? If you follow my advice I don't believe so. I cannot give you a 100% guarantee but you can read success stories online and I have thousands that I have counseled personally who succeeded.

You can be the next success story if you follow my advice! My goal is to help you get what you desire in life and right now he is it. Let's make that happen together!

Can We Just Be Friends?

"There comes a time in your life when you have to choose to turn the page, write another book or simply close it." — Shannon L. Adler

Now is the time to be strong and allow him to come back voluntarily into your life. And then you still need to be strong and not allow him total access to your love and adoration until he deserves it. You cannot be just friends with someone you have been intimately involved with until the intense feelings you have for that person subside. Trying to force a friendship will only backfire on you if you do it too soon.

If he were a close friend I don't think he would be willing to just walk away from you. After all, it takes quite a dramatic scenario for you to turn your back on your best friend or *soulmate.* So you must ask yourself if you were truly friends to begin with, and only you know the answer to that question. I know your boyfriend, husband or mate should be your best friend but frequently I find that it is just not the case.

Did he lie to you? Cheat on you? Abuse you emotionally or physically? If you answer is yes then he wasn't really a friend at all. Why would you expect him to suddenly be your friend after a break-up? Sometimes you must make the difficult decision to move on and this may be one of those times. You aren't playing mind games with him but you are keeping your sanity. Women who have strong personal boundaries are more likely to recover from a break-up than those who allow the man to make all the decisions. For instance, if he suggests you become friends because he isn't interested in an intimate relationship with you.

I can tell you that if he only wants to be friends while he is out on the town chasing women and sharing details with you he isn't interested in a relationship – with you. It is much easier and less hurtful for you to make the decision to move on and break all ties. Just the act of withdrawing from a man who was interested in you at one time can make him chase you again. He hates to lose something and the fear of loss is very motivating. You will become a challenge and men love challenges.

Are you really willing to be that girl he calls when another woman has broken his heart? I certainly hope not! If he is so detached that he has broken up with you then you can believe that he is open to finding a woman he considers more suitable. I use my relationship in examples because during our long-term relationship we have experienced just about every situation imaginable. An example: He confessed after we got back together that one of the reasons he walked away was that he felt could find someone more perfect and suitable for him than I. I laughed when he told me because it is humorous that men still believe there is a perfect relationship out there. The fact that he didn't see me as perfect didn't phase me because I love myself and am perfectly happy with who I am as a person.

Had we been "friends" during our time apart I would most likely have ended up hating his guts. I would not have wanted to subject myself to hearing about his online dating, sleepovers and *more perfect* women. I would have lost it and become a raving lunatic and certainly we would have never gotten back together. I don't know about you but I can only take so much rejection and then I snap. So thankfully I follow my own advice that I am sharing with you and I did not become his friend.

I had plenty of time to fall apart on my own and without him observing my sadness and despair. Yes, I allowed myself to stay in bed all day if I wanted but I didn't do it too often. In fact, I found hundreds of ways to keep busy so I didn't focus on him or the loss of my relationship. He never knew if I was upset, if I missed him or what was going on in my life or in my head. In his mind I was out partying with friends and other men. That's the vision I wanted him to have so not being friends with him was perfect!

If it doesn't work out that he comes banging down your door and you get over the intense feelings you can always reconnect and become friends. In fact, the no contact rule goes away if you no longer care about him or want him back. Just be sure you are totally over him before you get in touch. If you are fooling yourself you will know immediately because you will be back to the hot mess you were when you first broke up. You don't want that!

One more thing, when you want to be friends he knows he is still in control. He dumped you and you care enough that you will take the crumbs of a friendship rather than lose him totally. It is a ruse to get him to stay in touch and he knows it! He has the perfect scenario if you are friends. He can most likely get laid when he wants to as he uses you for a "friends with benefits" sidekick or confidante and he can also date other women. I don't think so! You should never be a back-up plan!

Ignore him, walk away and let him know you will be okay without him and watch him re-think things sooner or later. In fact, in a week or so you may consider sending him a goodbye letter to end things completely. Not a long, boring, heartfelt plea disguised as a goodbye letter but a real goodbye "don't let the door hit you in the ass" letter written with detachment and style. Certainly not a letter that implies you still want to be friends.

My suggestion is to say something like:

"It is my desire to end things and bring closure to our relationship because I think it is in both of our interests. I will miss _____ (a short description of something special you shared with him) but I wish you nothing but happiness, health and peace. Take care of yourself."

Short, sweet and to the point. When you do that and do not expect a response, reconciliation, or a plea from him, it will place you in control of your relationship. It is important in the healing phase to have some control over the outcome. You do that when you make the final break. Do not let that statement put fear in your heart that he will never contact you again. If he desires a relationship with you he will contact you! A simple letter will not stop him if he wants you back so don't be afraid to do it.

You have just thrown him off guard because that is totally different than his expectation of what would happen. No begging, no pleading, no stalking, no pushing you away? Just a simple, straightforward letter wishing him the best and saying goodbye? What the hell happened? His impression just went from negative to positive in his viewpoint of you. You have shown class and style and most of all independence. No talk of being sorry about what happened or just being friends to hold onto him. Just goodbye and good luck. Adios!

When you do something out of character you are gaining his interest. You are not the person he left. You have changed dramatically in a short amount of time. Does he want to meet the new you? Over time I believe he will. At first he may be in shock and he may wait to see if what he expected to happen will eventually happen. You chasing him! Don't let it happen! Move on and make new friends. His friendship has been replaced with other friendships – male and female.

Eventually you will make it a point to put yourself into his life through coincidences but right now you just go out with others. Date and have fun! I don't mean have sex with others unless you want to. That's an option. But keeping busy and dating others is a self-esteem building exercise that will keep you busy and positive about your life. During my breakups I made new BFFs (male and female) and they are still lifelong friends today.

My philosophy is that men may come and go but friends and family are forever. That doesn't mean that I don't have love and expectations from my lovers but it does mean that I don't place all my eggs in their one basket. Most women have experienced the fickle behavior of men and you realize that to have a full life you must have friendships outside of your mate's. Now is the time to renew old friendships and make new ones! Your life won't be empty if you do not place 100% of your happiness quotient on one person – the now "ex". Keep other relationships strong or develop new ones!

I find many times that the person I am counseling has allowed other relationships to wither and they have placed all of the responsibility for their happiness on their mate. Not only is that unhealthy but it is also unwise. Too much power and pressure placed on the other person can weigh them down until they want out of the pressure cooker. I do not want the responsibility for someone's happiness and I don't want another person to have to be my savior either.

Is He Worth The Effort?

"Sometimes it takes a heartbreak to shake us awake & help us see we are worth so much more than we're settling for." -- Mandy Hale

I haven't always chosen the right person for a variety of reasons. But the most likely reason is that whatever frame of mind I am in attracts the person I end up with. For instance, I am the "party girl" because I am going through a stage of rebellion and independence due to a recent breakup. Whom do I attract? It is the guy who resonates with the energy of freedom, fun and independence. Is that what I want long term? No! Or, I am feeling sad and lonely so what type of man do I attract? Perhaps one who is needy and smothers me with his insecurity.

Why am I writing about whether he is worth your time, energy and effort? Because sometimes we settle for what we have attracted and that person may not be our best possible choice. I find frequently that the more time we spend with someone who isn't Mr. Right the more time we waste trying to make him the right person. You must really look inside, deep inside, and determine whether you are settling for someone or choosing someone.

So many times I find that women settle for much less than they deserve in relationships. A man can treat you like a princess and get you hooked on that feeling before making a 180 degree turn and showing you his true colors. Rather than walk away a lot of women will spend too much time trying to change him back into the person they fell in love with, only to find out they were never really that person. It was a façade all along but many women never figure that out! My hot *soulmate* Allen turned out to be a hot mess and I have kept in touch with him a little over the years so I know he's never changed.

We all know women who pretend to be someone else when there is a man within hearing distance. They become flirtatious, coy or a vixen. Men do the same thing! They know the things that woman desire and they put them out there in conversations and actions as bait and women bite every time. For instance, men know that probably 99% of women want commitment. Whether it's a marriage or just commitment women want to know they have someone they can count on. I know numerous men who are lifelong bachelors but they allow the woman of the hour to believe she will be "the one" that makes him commit. She will be that amazing, special person that will change his mind. But he knows she isn't all the while leading her on to believe she is!

So, my question to you is whether your man is worth your time and energy. Has he been honest with you and stated that he only wants to be friends only to have you deny facts and continue to pressure him into something more? Is he a playboy who doesn't hide his alter ego but you stay with him hoping he will change? Has he cheated on you but you choose to believe it was one time only behavior that will never happen again? Is he open and honest with you or do you find that frequently he goes into "no contact" mode for no apparent reason placing doubts in your mind? Has he told you directly or indirectly that you are not the one and he wants to continue looking? Has he ever shown a temper or a controlling personality to the point you fear for your safety?

Women ignore signs the man she is devoted to is not the man she will conquer. Signs are there for a reason and you should always pay attention to them. If he is just killing time with you there will be obvious ways he will show you he has no intention of a long-term relationship. You will not be invited to family events, holiday parties or friend get-togethers. You will be a woman who is basically hidden from people who are important to him. You will not be a priority in his life and his focus will be only on what pleases him and makes him happy. He will make plans with you only to change them when a "better" offer comes along. He will come up with one excuse after another as he shows you are not a priority.

I am not telling you to be hyper sensitive about every move your mate makes, but I am saying you need to listen to what he says and pay attention to what he does. It will show you whether he is worth your time and effort. I wish I had counted all of the thousands of emails I have gotten from readers who want to know how they can change someone's mind about the relationship. Upon further review I usually find there were signs early in the relationship that it would be short-lived but the signs were ignored.

If a man wants a "friends with benefits" relationship and you don't want to settle for that you should be upfront and honest about it. Don't think you can eventually change his mind but until then you will allow your body to be used by him. I have dated many men in my lifetime and I am always honest with them and if I don't think they have what I am looking for then I don't date them – at all! Not even one date!

It may sound harsh but my time is precious to me and it is the only thing I can't replace. I want an honest, real, committed relationship and I am not interested in dating a man who wants a warm bed occasionally. I would rather sleep alone than be with someone incompatible. If a man doesn't show interest in me or give me what I desire I don't stick around hoping to change him or change his mind. I have too much independence and respect for myself to allow it.

Only you know whether he is worth your effort but I hope you determine the answer before you spend more time on getting him back. Don't let the fear of being without him or of being alone be the deciding factor. It is better to be alone than to be abandoned, used or abused. Most women believe that love is a feeling but there is more to it than that. Love is actually something that happens over time but it has nothing to do with the amount of time you spend with someone.

You should be able to list all of the reasons you love someone by listing their positive character traits. For instance:

- He is dependable and honest

- He is loving and considerate

- He exhibits respect for others as well as for you

- He keeps his word and you know you can count on him to be there for you

- He is honorable in every way

- He has real and meaningful conversations with you and you confide in each other

- He doesn't play games or intentionally hurt you

- He has an open heart and is willing to commit

- He is an open book and you never fear he would cheat, lie or hide anything from you

When you have a man whom I just described you know he is a quality man and I can see why he would mean the world to you. These are qualities that allow you to love someone. But you can see that love is not the "feeling" of wanting to have a sexual relationship or the dramatic feeling of "I can't live without them" regardless of how you are treated. It is a list of qualities that lead to an endearment of the person. Begin to look for that and less for the emotional attachment without justification and you won't be disappointed.

First step, decide whether he is worth it before proceeding to getting him back. Yes? Let's do it!

First Contact and How You Handle It

"Can officially confirm that the way to a man's heart these days is not through beauty, food, sex, or alluringness of character, but merely the ability to seem not very interested in him." — Helen Fielding

You know eventually you are going to "accidentally" run into him and you need to be prepared for the inevitable. What do you do? Being standoffish isn't going to work because it will turn him off totally. Ignoring him would be harmful to you and him. So what do you do and how do you act? The best way is to act as if you know him but you are not especially interested. Like if you were sitting next to someone at a bar and, while you find the person amusing, you don't go out of your way to connect with him or her.

During one of my breakups with my significant other I ran into him at an upscale bar I frequent. He and I were both totally shocked at the site of the other and I felt like bursting into tears. At the time it had been a few weeks that I had no contact with him and I was still raw. Not so upset that I stayed at home obviously, but definitely not ready for an encounter with him. I didn't prepare for the accidental meeting but I handled it the same way I suggest you handle it when you run into your "ex".

I turned around just as he and a male friend walked into the bar and, although we both looked surprised, we smiled and nodded to each other. He walked over and said hello to my girlfriend and I and I acted the same as I would with any stranger who was being friendly. I smiled and said hello and asked how he was doing. Nothing intimate at all. He said fine. How was I? "I'm great", I said with a smile. He said I looked beautiful as always and I thanked him. I asked him whether or not he saw my car parked in front because I had left my car with the valet and they always park it in front of the door. He said he had. I smiled and nodded which was my way of saying I didn't appreciate him coming into the place when he knew I was there.

I didn't ask him to sit down, have a drink or pay for mine. He stood there for a minute and said it was good to see me. I said thank you and turned back around to my friend and my drink. Granted I burst into tears the minute he left but I was totally in control and cool as a cucumber while in his presence. It perplexed him and it gave me an advantage. I looked good, I seemed happy, I was out having fun and it was clear that I had moved on. That's what you want, too.

When you run into him he will be expecting you to look longingly into his eyes, desperately trying to parlay the conversation into a longer exchange or lose your cool totally. That's not the way you need to behave around him. You need to be cool, friendly in a non-personal way, and a little aloof and mysterious. Like when you sit next to some stranger and you are friendly but you don't start jabbering about your cats at home, your horrible job or your lonely life.

After you have gone through a period of time with no contact and no stalking you will be able to return to the places where you know he may show up. Don't begin to hang out at places intentionally where he is likely to be because it will be too obvious. However, there will most likely be places you both loved and you aren't going to give them up because you are no longer together. Go there with a friend or a group of people and have fun. Not fake fun! Real fun! Without him!

If you have read any of my first three best selling books you will know about John. He was a love of mine and we enjoyed going to places together that I still go to. He stopped going because he cannot handle running into me but I continue to go there. When I do invariably I will run into friends of his. They are better friends to me now than they are to him but they always speak to me about him. That's what we have in common. I don't pry information out of them and I don't really care what he is doing so I don't continue the conversation in that direction. I know they go back to him and tell him that they have seen me but, because I don't have interest in what he is doing, they can't report back that I inquired about him.

That's what I want you to do. If you see his friends do not try to find out what he is doing, who he is dating, etc. They will ask about the two of you and when they do tell them briefly that you broke up and then change the subject. The fact that you are not actively seeking to find out about him will get back to him. Talk about anything else and make sure it is lighthearted and not serious. Have fun, laugh and enjoy yourself when you are out! What will happen when he sees his friends? How will the conversation go?

"I saw your ex-girlfriend the other night."

"Oh really, that's good. How is she?"

"Great! She was with some friends and they were partying and having fun."

He won't get feedback that you were drilling the person about your "ex". You weren't trashing him and telling them what an asshole he was. You didn't go into details about the breakup or ask about him. Wow! What happened? He will wonder if you have moved on already. He will have the vision of you out having fun with friends, being hit on by single men and having a blast. No thoughts of him at all? That will bother him much more than if you showed interest in what he was doing or how he was.

What if the first contact is through a text message? He sends a lame message to test the temperature of your response. Usually this will be short and noncommittal and is not intended to be anything of substance. He just wants to see if you are still there as a backup player. Your response should never be immediate and it should never be more than you have received. For instance, if he sends a simple "how are you" please do not respond with a novel or a tearful emoji. Your response may be with a simple "great" or even with an emoji thumbs-up or smiley face. But do not respond quickly.

Also, I would respond erratically. Sometimes you may respond and sometimes you may not. Or you may respond to every second or third message. You are no longer together and you don't need to drop what you are doing to jump when he wants you to jump. You're busy! You are having fun, on a date, out with friends, or perhaps you just forgot he sent a message. He is no longer the center of your world and you shouldn't treat him as if he were.

I would be friendly, funny and brief. In the beginning of my relationship with my man I was dating others and I didn't know if I wanted him to be my one and only. He would fake butt dial me and put the phone in his pocket so I could hear that he was out talking to people, listening to music and possibly on a date. I would send a brief text saying something like "better watch out I may hear something I shouldn't" or something insignificant and flirtatious. Before you text back I want you to think lighthearted thoughts and respond accordingly.

I received one text message that said, "Better make up your mind about me because these women are chasing me and they may catch me first". I responded "run Forrest run" or something stupid. But I didn't text him first and I took my time to respond to his messages. Sometimes I would wait a day or two before responding but they were always lighthearted. We were just beginning to date and I wasn't going to be chosen by him – I was going to choose him after careful deliberation. Men are accustomed to being in control of the relationship but it is time that women get used to it, too.

If you jump into a serious discussion with him he will bolt so keep your interactions light. No heavy discussions, accusations, apologies or crying allowed. The tone you set when you first have contact will determine the outcome of the breakup and how fast you get him back. If you decide you want him back! After you have used my guided meditations to empower yourself and cut the cord that binds you together with him you may decide you can do better than a guy who walks away without provocation. You deserve a man who loves, adores and is totally committed to you. Keep your distance and your cool and if indeed he is "the one" he will knock down any obstacle to making that happen.

Time To Get Serious!

"If a girl starts out all casual with a guy and she doesn't tell him that she wants a relationship, it will never become a relationship. If you give the guy the impression that casual is okay with you, that's all he'll ever want. Be straight with him from the start. If he gets scared and runs away, he wasn't right for you." -- **Sussane Colasanti**

I realize that many of you have already made this mistake with your man when you pretended that casual was okay with you because you were hoping he would want more after realizing how wonderful you were. Although it didn't work out the way you envisioned it is not too late to change it. You are now in the process of getting your man back but when he does return you need to ask yourself if you are going to be satisfied with continuing your relationship without commitment.

I have mentioned that it is not what I want nor would it be what I would accept from a mate. I let them know that upfront but many women don't want to risk losing the man by stating what she desires. Now is the time to look into your heart and acknowledge what it is that you really, really want in a relationship. If it is commitment then you will not accept less. You can still make a stand and get what you desire from the "ex" but you must make him the one who puts the handcuffs on his own wrists.

After one entire year of no contact with my partner he proposed within 3 weeks of our reconciliation. We had been together for 4 years before our separation and his casual attitude about our relationship was one of the reasons we split up. How did I get him to propose? I didn't give him an ultimatum when we resumed our relationship but I let him know that I was not interested in continuing our relationship and wasting my time because he obviously just wanted a playmate.

I allowed him the opportunity to pursue me and convince me that he really wanted to spend the rest of his life with me. I wasn't willing to have him back again under his conditions. I had conditions of my own and I needed to honor them. I had inadvertently presented myself to be so independent and accepting that I was willing to be kept on hold for an indefinite period of time while allowing him to call all the shots. I wasn't willing to do that anymore and he was immediately made aware of that fact.

What had changed? Well, in the beginning of our relationship I was in a different mindset and, as I mentioned earlier, whatever you project you will attract. I was newly single and ready to mingle and it was okay that this man was known as a playboy of sorts. The problem is that over time I returned to my normal self but I had attracted an opposite man whom I now loved. That turned out to be a major obstacle in our relationship. He said all the right things but his actions proved that he was coasting through our relationship and would have been content to continue as long as I would let him.

I expressed to him my desires before the breakup and he responded by saying we were too different and he set off on his own to find that *perfect* woman. In hindsight it was actually healthy for our relationship. You cannot force someone to change but you can get them to change on their own. Since it was his idea to get back together and it was his idea to propose to me he didn't feel manipulated or trapped. I had simply stated that although I still cared for him we were too different and I wanted something more than he wanted. That simple fact made him realize that he wanted me more than he wanted his freedom.

So even though I didn't tell him from the "get-go" that I was a one-man-woman who expected monogamy and commitment -- it wasn't too late to change the outcome. My point of telling you my story is because if you *JUST* want your "ex" back into your life, without changing, you may end up getting exactly the same person who left. If you were happy with that then bless you and your union! However, if you want something more from him now is the time to make him step up and be the person you need in your life. I have readers who are so focused on getting their man to return they don't realize that it didn't work out before and it may be unlikely to work out again. Changes need to be made in order to stay together.

I find that frequently commitment is a big hurdle and it can be the reason for the breakup in the first place. You want more and he wants less. If that is the case when he pursues you again you should explain to him why it would not work. Men love to convince you that they are worthy, especially if they are competing against someone else. Your argument would not be "you must commit" but rather something less intimidating like "I know you enjoy your freedom and I am ready for a relationship that can lead to permanency". In other words, we are worlds apart in our goals and desires. Let him know that you are open to having someone wonderful sweep you off your feet but you aren't going to settle for less than you deserve.

I know a woman who wants to get married and it doesn't matter whom she marries. She just searches for men who may be available to fulfill her desire to be taken care of financially. You aren't that woman! You want a relationship with a man who desires the same things in life that you desire. You aren't trying to trap a man into marriage because you're needy or are tired of working and need an extra paycheck. You needs are important so be upfront, honest and forthright about them. Remember, men must be available physically and emotionally, have the ability to be a committed relationship, be able to be your best friend that you can count on and be your spiritual equal. Find that in a mate and you can be happy and content forever.

The thought that expressing your desires and wants may chase him off for good may frighten the living hell out of you and I understand. But you must decide whether you are willing to give up yourself to be what he wants or whether you would be willing to risk a loss for ultimate happiness. I can't answer that question for you. If you're willing to keep things casual and hope he commits after a period of time then let your conscience guide you. If you want your man to be different then you need to treat him differently.

What does that mean? No more casual sex hoping for a deep and meaningful connection. Billy Crystal said it best – "Women need a reason to have sex and men just need a place." Sex without intimacy and commitment is not very fulfilling emotionally. There is no judgment call on my statement because it is just a fact. I have a friend who has slept with literally thousands of men! She admits it and I don't pass judgment on her or else I wouldn't be her friend. She recently got married and after her nuptials she called me and very innocently said "He is the only man who has ever kissed me during sex". Her statement shocked me so I asked what she had experienced with other men. She said they were all about the sexual act but not about the connection. It was literally the "wham, bam, thank you ma'am" encounter.

She had sex with many men but there was no connection and no real intimacy. She didn't even know what she was missing until she finally met a man who fell in love with her. Sex doesn't make the man fall for you – it makes you fall for the man. Why? Because there is a natural chemical released in your brain called Oxytocin that is literally a feel good love drug. When the chemical is released it is a mood elevator that causes you to feel emotionally attached to the person you are having sex with.

Normally that is not a bad thing but there is no discernment about the person you are in bed with so he could be a real "bad boy" and you will still have the positive feelings. If you have an "ex" that you feel you can win back through a hot sexual exchange all it will do is make you even more attached. Stay away from intimacy until you have what you desire from the relationship! Tell him what you want from a relationship and either he will step up and give you what you want, negotiate for a compromise or walk away. If he walks away he was not the right one for you! Rather than spend countless weeks, months or even sometimes years pining over him you must then move on.

I cannot tell you the number of times men have left for long periods of time only to return and want the woman back. I don't want you to put your life on hold hoping for this outcome but it is a definite possibility. Whether he does or not the next relationship you are in promise yourself not to hold back your wants, needs and desires from the person. Be honest about what you are looking for and if he is not the person to fulfill your needs then move on. Be strong and decisive!

New Confident YOU!

"It is of practical value to learn to like yourself. Since you must spend so much time with yourself you might as well get some satisfaction out of the relationship." -- Norman Vincent Peale

My life's purpose has been to help women in all areas of their lives. I have found that low self-esteem causes a plethora of problems for women all over the world. You cannot have a low opinion of yourself and attract a mate who will see you in higher regard than you see yourself. You absolutely must love yourself, like yourself and honor yourself! I remember at one point in my life where I thought that self-love was a narcissistic action and it did not appeal to me. I was not accustomed to putting myself first and I found that I had to really work on it. That is no longer the case thank goodness.

Since you cannot escape the person you are I suggest that if you have what you consider faults or deficits in your character or personality that you work to improve those areas. In fact, I have created numerous guided meditations available only on my website designed to empower women in all areas of their lives. I believe that unless you learn to appreciate yourself you are likely to end up in meaningless relationships with the wrong person. The higher the self-esteem the less likely you are to end up wasting precious time convincing someone you really are a person worth their love. You will learn to rely less on the approval of others and more on your own wonderful inner guidance system.

It never ceases to amaze me that so many women just hand over the control of their lives to a man who is unworthy. If you understand that it is because you feel less than you should feel about yourself you can take a step to change your direction. We all have friends in relationships where we wonder what the hell they are doing with such losers. We clearly see they are worthy and deserving of so much more than they settle for and it frustrates us that we cannot get their worthiness across to them. And, sometimes we are that person that our friend's look at and wonder what the hell are we thinking. It goes both ways!

If nothing more comes from this book than getting you to sit down and list your wonderful qualities while admiring the person you are it will be worth it. You see when someone really likes and loves who they are they aren't going to fall into a relationship where they are treated poorly. When you look into the mirror and care about the person looking back at you there will be a change in you. You will no longer waste away in a sea of Kleenex and empty ice cream containers or Vodka bottles over your breakup, you will wonder what the hell the idiot "ex" was thinking when he left. Is he nuts?

If you place your value on someone else's opinion you may always be disappointed. How many people build up others regardless of their affection for them? Not many! Too often men and women will tear down your image in order to make themselves appear better. I have a friend who is just absolutely drop dead gorgeous. I mean she is a complete beauty inside and outside. Other friends never compliment her, however. In fact, they do just the opposite. They pay compliments to our mutual friends who are plain Jane's and ignore this friend's stunning beauty. Why? Because by doing that I believe they think she will be taken down a notch. Although she is beautiful her self-esteem is tied to their approval. She has no idea how lovely she is and that's so sad.

When you work on your confidence not only does it enhance your beauty it will allow you to shine without the approval of others. The relationship you have with yourself will shape all of your other relationships whether they are friends or lovers. Even if you are not a beauty like my friend, and there aren't too many of us that are, you will have a confidence and radiance that will attract others like a magnet.

I talk a lot about your subconscious mind in my other books so I won't go into great detail in this one except to say that your subconscious mind is approximately 10,000 times more powerful than your conscious mind. So whatever you tell yourself in your inner mind – that self-talk that we do constantly throughout the day – resonates within at a deep level that has the ability to change your life. Whether it is positive or negative it has the ability to be imbedded in a way that will direct our lives without our even knowing it.

How can we love or even like ourselves and create the person we desire to be? And, is it necessary? Yes! One of the best ways to change your attitude about yourself, improve your health, create confidence, lose weight, empower yourself, control your relationship and your mate is to meditate. I know a lot of readers may not meditate or even know what it is but it can change your life. Meditation is a deep, regenerating type of relaxation that gets you in touch with your powerful subconscious mind. It has the ability to change even your health and self-esteem. Also, it allows you to mentally communicate with your "ex" and others and it is one of the most powerful things you can do to get him back.

I have little self-talk affirmations that I do throughout the day for a few minutes. I also meditate but I don't always have time to do a full meditation during the day. My abbreviated method allows my brain to tell my body what it desires. For instance, I tell my body that every cell in it is perfect in every way, I am healthy and beautiful, I am strong and confident, and I create my future and attract wonderful things to me every moment of every day. For some that may sound like gibberish but trust me it works like magic!

Focus just for a moment on any part of your body and tell it to relax. You can feel that thought is energy and when you direct it your body will respond. It is the same thing you will do for a little self-love. Tell yourself that you love yourself, you are a wonderful person, and a generous person deserving only beautiful things and you will direct a different future for yourself. Meditation, affirmations and mental reminders of your worth throughout the day will create a stronger and more powerful woman. The more powerful and in control of your life you are the less you will be misdirected by others.

I am such a believer in the Law of Attraction and creating the life you desire that I recorded guided meditations for my readers and they are on my website at http://laniestevensauthor.com. I tell you this not because I get rich from them but because they are the easiest and best way to tap into your subconscious, creative mind. Once you learn to really value yourself and what you have to offer in a relationship you will not be tempted to settle for someone who cannot or will not give it to you.

I want you to take a moment and close your eyes to visualize your "ex". See him as perfectly as you can in your mind's eye. You may be able to sense him, see him, smell him or just imagine that you are. Allow your heart area to open up and relax as you visualize him in as much detail as possible. Imagine that you are sending him love, forgiveness and gratitude for the time you spent together. See a connection going from your heart area to his connecting the two of you. It is a silver or gold or pink glowing cord that attaches you. Now just mentally send love to him before disconnecting.

In my "Pussy Whip" book I give you details on how to connect and control your mate but I just want you to take a few moments to realize that you can connect just through the power of your subconscious mind. I won't write 112 pages about the method, because it is in my other books, but I just want to point out the ability you have to visualize. If you see yourself as weak, unworthy and a victim you will become that person. If you visualize yourself as strong, independent, worthy and a prize you will become that person. Never see yourself as that person you do not desire to be!

He Wants To See You!

"Forgiveness does not change the past, but it does enlarge the future." -- Paul Boose

Okay, you've moved on with your life hopefully. You have increased your self-worth immensely by the power of your thoughts and actions, you aren't willing to settle for less than you desire, you are dating and having fun – you are a new, improved version of your former self. But, you still care about that pesky "ex" and you plan to see him. Hopefully you will be strong and not allow him to run the relationship as he did before. You are now ready to meet him and allow him to convince you to give him another shot OR you are ready to stay single and attract an even better match.

You would never even dream of contacting him but he has reached out to you for a date or a meeting and you agree. Most often this is what will happen but occasionally he will not contact you for a prolonged period of time. If that happens you will know that he is either a stubborn ass or he is just not interested in reconnecting with you. Either way you have to let it be okay with you because you no longer look to him, or anyone else, to confirm your desirability.

If he does want to meet you must be strong and firm in your conviction. What does that mean? Don't jump at the offer to meet with high expectations or an immediate response that implies you are chomping at the bit to see him. In fact, don't agree to meet with him right away. Without going into detail about the reason I want you to casually say you would love to meet later in the week. Suggest another time to see him but don't say why or that you are "busy". The fact that you aren't available will make him curious about whether there is another man but don't confirm or deny it.

If you decide to see him don't let him come to your house to pick you up. Suggest a convenient place to meet him. You are starting a new relationship with him and you aren't just picking up where the old relationship left off. A neutral place lets you arrive and leave when you desire. Don't overstay your welcome! You should be the first to leave and the first to hang-up the phone should there be a phone call. Don't hang on his every word and let him end the meeting or the phone call – you do it! Leave him wanting more of you and not wondering how soon he can escape.

Don't get drunk and drool all over him at a bar or allow him to come back to your house for casual sex. Treat him as if he were a new match.com date. You can flirt with him at a distance, tease him playfully and cutely but you aren't going further than that. If he wants to talk about your breakup that's fine but don't talk about all the negative details. Yeah, it happened and you are over it should be the attitude you have so you don't need to persuade him of the fact. Even if he tells you that he is dating someone new or that you will never get back together you must act cool, calm and collected.

Remember – don't make someone a priority when you are simply an option! If he is simply bored and half interested and all he wants to do is pass the time don't hang around. The fact that he has disappeared from your life and now reappears shouldn't make you jump back into the relationship. Being fickle doesn't create trust between the two of you so make sure he really wants more with you before committing to even trying again.

I know you fear him walking away for good but you survived after the breakup and you will survive should that happen. Worse than having him disappear again is letting him lead you on with empty promises or playing with your emotions. Set strong personal boundaries and don't allow game playing! Being the one to withdraw from the encounter may make him chase you again if he is interested. He may try to regain control by being distant and aloof. That's fine! It is only to gain control of you and have you draw closer and do what he wants you to do. If that happens thank him for the dinner, drink or time and leave!

If your fear of loss is too great you may find you will desire to chase him. Do not under any circumstances chase a man who has dumped you. If you meet him for a date it is not okay for you to discuss your future, whether there is a future, the past or anything negative. No snide comments or sadness. You are a new woman and you cannot allow him to throw you off guard even for a second. And, he may try when he senses that you have changed. He may test the waters by making statements he knows will hurt you. Things like how much fun he has been having, a trip he went on, dating websites, parties or functions where you would question if he were alone.

If that happens do not interrogate him. Let the statements pass as if they don't matter at all. "Really? That sounds like fun." That's all you need to say then change the subject. Don't ask who was on the trip, how many women were at the party or whether he has met anyone online. If he asks about your personal life give him the short version with no details and change the subject. The best way to change the subject is to ask a neutral question. Or bring up something totally unrelated but act as if the thought was triggered by his questions.

At the end of the meeting or "date" thank him and tell him it was good to see him. Kiss his cheek if it seems appropriate or let him be the first to make a move to hug you. No intimacy at all! Don't gaze at him like he is a 16-ounce filet mignon either! He's a man who broke your heart and he needs to step up and prove he is worthy to even get another date with you. Do not text him or contact him after your date. If he wants to contact you he will. If not, keep up your social life and you may even step it up a little!

You aren't holding onto negative feelings and anger over what happened between you and your "ex". In fact, you have forgiven him and yourself for the breakup. You were both most likely responsible in some way. Forgiveness and the ties that bind you together through anger and bitterness are unhealthy and it's important that you dismiss them. He will be able to feel the release of energy as well as see it in your eyes. The energy of hate, anger and betrayal are very heavy and uninviting. Release them for your own well-being and health.

The man loved you at one time and seeing you as you were when you met, when he first became infatuated with you, will ignite feelings within him whether he shows it or not. Just having you be the sweet, forgiving, wonderful woman he fell in love with is going to be such a relief for him it will open up his heart to you. And that is true whatever the outcome of the meeting turns out to be. There is no need to be anything but kind to him and that act alone will show him that you are not holding onto the past or to a grudge. It will prove that you have truly moved past the pain.

"Forgive the past. It is over. Learn from it and let go. People are constantly changing and growing. Do not cling to a

limited, disconnected, negative image of a person in the past. See that person now. Your relationship is always alive and changing." – Brian L. Weiss

A Future Together

"Some of the biggest challenges in relationships come from the fact that most people enter a relationship in order to get something: they're trying to find someone who's going to make them feel good. In reality, the only way a relationship will last is if you see your relationship as a place that you go to give, and not a place that you go to take." – Anthony Robbins

Taking your steps slow and easy allows you to see whether he will begin to give you what you need in order for the relationship to survive. It's easy in the throes of passion and missing someone to make promises that you may not be able to keep. You have decided through careful analysis that he is definitely the love of your life but you also need to make sure that you are his. It cannot be a one-way relationship or it will never last and never be fulfilling. After all, a relationship that lasts is a true give-and-take between two committed people.

I know many people who are only looking for someone to give them something in the form of security, companionship or simply a warm body. They are not in tune with the other person enough to know what they need or how to give it to them. Some men need nothing more than love and a peaceful environment. I have a male friend who states that "being needed" by someone is the most important thing in a relationship. Whatever that special thing is we are seeking the other person needs to be made aware of it. A relationship that lasts rarely is one where you find someone who just makes you feel good – all the time!

If you have found yourself to always be the giver in the relationship and the other person is the taker obviously changes need to be made. Ideally a 50/50 relationship would be what we would end up with but that is never the case. There are times when you must give 100% when the other person isn't able and they reciprocate with 100% when you are unable to give. But when you consistently find you are giving more and more and it is never enough it is time to stop giving at all. Move on!

I sincerely hope you have gotten back together in a mutually beneficial manner and he is more than willing to commit to you. Too often people get back together under the same conditions as the ones where they split-up and it is easy to see that it will not last because no changes were made. You have hopefully made huge strides to empower yourself, strengthen your resolve, list the non-negotiable items, raised your vibration and self-esteem through meditation and affirmations and are ready for your new and improved "ex" to be back in your life.

You must remember that while you have gone through a transformation he has most likely done little soul searching or changing. It will be your responsibility to change your relationship through the changes you have made. By your behavior and acceptance or rejection of his treatment you will mold his reactions and your future. It is always up to us to determine how others treat us but now more than ever you must be aware of it. If he slips back into treating you disrespectfully or as though you are not a priority you must let him know it is unacceptable or walk away for good.

Getting the person back is only one part of the success. You may find that you have grown and he has remained the same selfish asshole he was when you were together before. Nothing changed except the time you wasted mourning his loss. I hope that isn't the case but if it is recognize it early and do something about it. Don't let yourself slip back into an unhealthy relationship where he controls your emotions and destiny. It is better to be alone than to be with the wrong person.

As if you were parenting a child you cannot allow him to get away with bad behavior or be inconsistent with your actions. When you get back together it is best to address the issues you know caused problems in the past and reach a resolution about how to handle them. My mate and I have issues with disagreements. We both disconnect when there is an issue and it is really unhealthy in the long term. We agreed that if one of us left (which we usually do) we would not allow more than 24 hours to pass before reconnecting in some manner. It has worked for us.

So whether it is anger issues, disconnecting, jealousy, commitment or any other problem you may have it must be addressed and resolved. Don't rehash the issue because it is in the past. Don't place blame or go on about the problems for hours and hours. Acknowledge there was a problem and it is extremely likely the same problem will recur. Come up with a solution that is acceptable by both parties while you are both calm and determined to make your relationship successful. It is much easier than trying to address it when you are in the throes of anger or rage.

Knowing that people don't fundamentally change is important to your success. If he had annoying habits in the past he hasn't magically gotten rid of them in your absence. You must accept him and not try to change him to meet your unique specifications. There are tons of things that drive me nuts and I have to bite my tongue to not mention them when I am in a bad mood or irritated. I watch my big mouth and my very telling body language for the most part. He can't help it if he smacks the hell out of gum and his popcorn. However, the important things that really matter are non-negotiable.

I will never, ever allow him to walk away for a friggin' year with no contact. In fact, he is very aware that if that happens again he is history with a capital H. I can see his wheels turning when we have a disagreement because he doesn't want to lose me and he is the first to reconnect when he has jumped into his car and sped off like an idiot. He changed not because he chose to do it but because I won't allow anything else. Let's just say I have been there and done that (as have you) and we aren't going to let that behavior slide anymore.

While having a relationship with someone we know and love is easier and more comforting in a strange way it is not a good reason to stay in a relationship that is one-sided or selfish. I have always been a giver and of course he was the taker. It is now quite even although it still may be that I am a little more of a giver than he is. But he has made great strides for a somewhat selfish male. Maybe one reason is that I have stopped acting like a wife when I am just the fiancé (and before that just the girlfriend). Unless you have a ring on your finger and a lifetime commitment you don't need to be a wife to your mate. If you act like a wife why does he need to marry you?

Be the best, most loving, kind, generous and wonderful woman you can be and if he doesn't appreciate it be willing and able to let him go. Usually when men see that you have enough love and respect for yourself that you will not tolerate bad or inconsistent behavior they will value you enough to straighten up their act. Occasionally that doesn't happen but if it doesn't you are strong enough, as you have already proven, to be on your own and creating a wonderful life for yourself. Don't stick around for long if when the honeymoon is over he returns to being the person you didn't like or respect.

It amazes me how many women put up with and accept bad behavior from men when there are so many good men out there. My suggestion to you if you decide to let the "ex" go is when you date again to be aware of signs from men that they are not the one and never will be. Let them go fast and don't waste a lot of time or make excuses for them. A friend of mine has never been dumped in her lifetime. Why? At the first sign of bad behavior on his part, or if he shows the slightest disinterest, she dumps him. According to her (and I agree) it is easier to get over someone if you are the one who walks away.

I truly believe you will be able to reconnect with your "ex" if you just follow the simple but effective steps I outlined. You want the man you love to respect and love you, be faithful and honest, care about your feelings and welfare and make you a priority in his life. If you require those things in your relationship AND give those things to him you will have a match made in heaven. I know how much you want him in your life but forsaking your own desires will eventually cause you to be miserable and end up in divorce court. Get him back on your terms and allow him to see that you can be happy without him because you are a woman who will never accept less than she deserves.

This list will remind you of things to do to regain control of your life, your mate and your happiness:

- Be open and honest about what you desire from your "ex" as well as all men

- Don't accept less than you deserve

- Choose the man and don't fall into a relationship because he chose you

- Use your imagination and visualization to create a life through the Law of Attraction

- Don't condone or accept behavior that is unacceptable

- Forgive him and yourself so you can heal

- Don't be too eager when he contacts you because when you are he will instinctively back away

- Keep your cool and set your goals for your relationship

- Use affirmations daily to strengthen your resolve, increase your self-esteem and empower your life

- Be willing to move on should he not live up to your expectations

- Stay busy and engaged with friends and dates

- Rejection is an opportunity for selection – don't settle!

- Remember, there are millions of men in the world so he isn't the best catch possible however much you may love him

I wish for you a long, happy relationship with your loved one and I have no doubts that will happen. Stay strong because you will never have what you desire through weakness. Many blessings to you!

Contact the Author

Lanie Stevens lives in Austin, Texas and spends her time writing, traveling and collecting experiences. I hope you will join the Law of Attraction forum to share your experiences using the advice in this book with other powerful women from all over the world.

Meditations:

http://laniestevensauthor.com

Forum:

http://laniestevensforum.boardhost.com

I hope you enjoyed the book! If you would take a moment to write a positive review it would really be appreciated! Thank you, sister!

Made in the USA
Middletown, DE
08 September 2019